Aromatherapy:

Easy Recipes For 100% Natural Deodorants And Mild Soap

Table of Content :

Book 1

Introduction 6

Chapter 1 – Why Deodorants Are Important? 7

Chapter 2 – Artificial Versus Natural Deodorants...14

Chapter 3 – Amazing All-Natural Deodorant Recipes 22

Conclusion 28

Book 2

Introduction: 31

Chapter 1 – Different Kinds of Soaps 32

Chapter 2 – Soap Recipes For Smoother Skin 44

Chapter 3 – DIY Germicidal Soap Recipes 48

Chapter 4 – Colorful Soap Recipes 51

Chapter 5 – Creative Multipurpose Soap Recipes 55

Conclusion 61

Debra Hill

Deodorants:

Easy Recipes For Fresh and Effective Deodorants

Deodorants:

Easy Recipes For Fresh and Effective Deodorants

Introduction

When I was still a child I am not experiencing any kinds of bad odor especially on my armpit, it was only when I reached my adolescent stage when I experienced a significant change especially on my metabolism. I began to sweat more which is really a great deal on why I accumulated a bad odor especially on my armpit since then. I was frustrated and helpless because I have no idea on what to do in battling my bad odor problem. It was really a nightmare for me because I was bullied and I cannot do anything because what they are saying are all true.

I asked my mom on what do I need to do to combat the problem. She told me that I have to cleanse carefully my body especially the armpit when I am taking a bath and apply a deodorant afterward. I did the routines that my mom advice throughout the years until I became an adult however I am noticing that it has a lot of side-effects not only my skin but also on my overall wellness.

This is the primary reasons why I discovered that the artificial deodorant that I am using is composed of chemicals that are harmful to the health. This is where I had an urge to learn how to make natural deodorant recipes for personal use.

It truly changed my life for the better because it made myself healthier and most importantly free from bad odor. As time passed by, I realized that it wasn't enough for me to keep the knowledge by myself so I decided to share it to you on this book so that you will also have the ability to enjoy the privilege that I have.

Chapter 1 – Why Deodorants Are Important?

Imagine a situation where you enter a public vehicle, let's say a bus or train, or let's say a public place, and then there you are, you suddenly hold your breath or covered your nose for long because of that unwanted smell roaming around the place? Of course, you know that it came from someone's sweaty underarms and then you might say that "do they even use deodorant?" We all know that it is embarrassing especially if we are on that person's place.

But did you know that the sweat our body produces is odorless or close to it? Then you might ask: "Then where did that bad smell came from?" So let's start with it, our skin pores in the body produce sweat because of the waste that passes through it. The hotter the climate is the more sweat our body produces especially on the warm parts of our bodies, like for example, the underarms.

The bad smell that we all hate doesn't come from the sweat, but from bacteria that is on the sweat. There are a lot of people that use deodorant, and some use them almost every day and continues it for a long period of time where stopping the use if it will never be an option. There are also other people who don't really need these deodorants or simply does not use them at all, and believe me it is all fine. But for those who use deodorants, they don't really know that the effectiveness of it is just low.

We all know that the deodorant's purpose is to get rid of the body odor in us. And yes it is the main reason and the only reason we have that's why we use deodorants. There is something like deodorant that is called "Antiperspirants", but they function differently. Antiperspirants keep us from producing body odor thus making us smell fresh, and they stop our sweat glands to produce too much sweat.

But take note that antiperspirants don't really work, I mean, like the deodorant, its effectiveness is low because there will be a time that our body will reject and become immune from the effects of the antiperspirant.

Like you, I am also curious about how exactly deodorants get rid of the bad smell our body have. In all honesty, both things, the deodorant, and antiperspirants are quite complicated. But here today, I'll be listing down some of the effects of deodorants on our body.

1. *Deodorants eliminate those odor-causing bacteria*

Like what I've just said earlier, sweat is almost completely odorless, because there are some studies that proved sweat is nearly odorless. Body odor comes out when the body's bacteria breaks down one of two types of sweat. That only means, the bad smell that we usually produce from excessive sweating doesn't come out right after we sweat for a small amount, and if the sweat doesn't stay too long from your skin. So all in all, the main idea of deodorant is that they can kill the bacteria that causes bad odor, and that is all.

2. *Deodorants do not stop you from sweating*

Well, the daily use of deodorants and antiperspirants led some of us to believe that they both work the same way but in reality, they don't. Just like said recently, deodorants keep us from smelling bad, they get rid of the bacteria in the sweat, but they don't stop the sweat glands from producing sweat.

Now, on the other hand, the antiperspirants help to stop the production of excess sweat on the sweat glands in order to get rid of excessive and unwanted sweat, especially on the underarms.

So to sum it all up, we put our money on the antiperspirants as they can help you get rid of this annoying extra sweat the same time maintain you smelling fresh, but do keep in mind that they only decrease the sweat glands production of sweat by only 20%.

3. Use of deodorant can change the bacteria in the body

There is a study that stated, the use of deodorants and antiperspirants can change the skin microbiome, meaning that they can somehow affect the bacteria in our body. In this study conducted, there were 17 persons where they are examined for about eight days. The researchers swabbed each of the person's underarms.

The first day of the study, the participants of the study does their standard underarm hygiene routine. Starting the second day up to the sixth, they all stopped using antiperspirants and deodorants. And for the last two days, the seventh and eighth, all of them applied antiperspirants.

As for the final result, it has shown that everyone who participated in the study has an increase of bacteria on their underarms the time they stopped using the antiperspirants and deodorants.

4. Use of deodorant can lead to breast cancer

Some might say that women who use deodorants and antiperspirants every day can increase the chances of them having breast cancer in the future. This may bother some of you, but here is an explanation of why it is not true. There is a theory that stated, the aluminum in the antiperspirants and the parabens in the deodorants can produce some hormonal effects, estrogen-like.

These things can contribute in the growth of breast cancer cells and there are a few numbers of scientific studies that stated there is somehow a connection, but the FDA and the National Cancer Institute does not support this claims.

Now knowing this, we think that you should not be afraid of using deodorants and antiperspirants, why? It is because it is not proven that it can lead to breast cancer, and there are no cases which stated they developed breast cancer because they use deodorants and antiperspirants daily. There are still studies being conducted about these claims, and as long as it is not yet proven, the use of these products are completely safe.

Why Deodorants are very important for Women in Modern Life?

The use of antiperspirants and deodorants are very high especially on hotter places on earth, for one good reason, people there sweat a lot. And we have our own lives, we have our own jobs, and things we do, physically to be exact, and because of this, we also sweat a lot, like a lot. So how to deal with it?

Grab your deodorant or antiperspirant and your good to go. Well, believe it or not, but these products, the antiperspirants, and deodorants have been running all along the way back to the time of the Ancient Egyptians, well actually it started from them.

They experiment with different natural materials to use as scented products for the underarms, one example is cinnamon. But here in our modern world, most antiperspirants and deodorants contain chemicals in order for a better and likable result.

A lot of us are annoyed when we sweat especially when you are working on an office or a place that is air-conditioned because when the bad odor starts to kick in, it will just spread out in the whole place and the smell will just stay there and somehow will leave a dark spot in your shirt near the underarms. It is just embarrassing, right? But you should know that sweating is actually good for the body.

Sweating is a normal thing that happens in the body, it is a natural way of cooling our bodies when it is hot. So come to think about what happens when you stop it. That is what happens every single time you use an antiperspirant. So it is still important to put the balance on things and try not to use them daily.

Well, having some knowledge about deodorants and antiperspirants can be good, but what if you process more info about it? Like for example, did you know that we spend almost $18 billion dollars a year for these products, just for the sake of removing bad odors or making your sweat glands stop producing sweat? Come think of that $18 billion dollars. And here, I'll be listing down some of the things that you might not know about antiperspirants and deodorants.

1. *Deodorant eliminates bacteria*

Well, we all know that the one that causes those bad odors are the bacteria on the sweat, right? So here is the deodorant coming up to save the day. They will keep you smelling good as they eliminate those bacteria that lies in your sweat.

2. *The anti-body odor is an old-time trend*

Yes, you heard that right. Like said from the previous one up there, the Ancient Egyptians made the first anti-body odor products which are later known as deodorants.

And did you know that the first ever trademarked deodorant is called Mum and was created in 1888, man that is a long time ago. And after 15 years, the first ever antiperspirant came out and it is called Everdry.

3. *Antiperspirants do not really stop the production of sweat.*

This aluminum found in antiperspirants does a good job of stopping the eccrine sweat glands. But it is just 20 percent effective.

4. *Your body can become immune to the antiperspirant you use daily*

Believe it or not but our bodies can adapt to the effects an antiperspirant can do to our sweat glands, and no one knows how can this happen. Some said that the body can find its own way of resisting the effects and starts to produce more sweat on other glands. A doctor said that it is better to have a variety of brands for deodorants and antiperspirants in order to prevent the body to adapt from its effects.

5. Whether you're a man or woman, deodorant is effective

Do you know that women have more sweat glands than men? Yes, it's true but the cool thing here is men's sweat glands produces more sweat then women do. Although there are separate products or brands of antiperspirants and deodorants that are specified for men and women, in reality, they are all the same, and all of these "separated" things is just a marketing strategy. And it is funny to think that all of us still falls for this kind of marketing. The only thing that differs is the style and scent of the deodorant.

6. *Some people do not need deodorants*

Well, some may advertise really well that people are still convinced to buy and use deodorants every day. And do you know that most people don't smell bad at all? Yes, it is all true. And some people are simply lucky because they naturally don't smell bad at all because of their genes.

7. *No one really knows where those yellow stains came from*

Not even the ones who make deodorants and antiperspirants and not even the scientists know why are there yellow stains left in the underarms when they use deodorants and antiperspirants.

But the main thing here is that some theorize that it came from the aluminum compounds which can be seen on antiperspirants as they have certain chemical reactions with the sweat, shirt or the skin. And according to some research, the best way to get rid of these yellow stains is just to simply avoid buying and using aluminum-based antiperspirants.

8. *You can produce your own deodorant and antiperspirant*

Isn't that amazing that you can improvise or somehow create your own deodorant and antiperspirant right at your own home! Well, there are certain things or ingredients needed in order to make one.

The bright side of making your own deodorant or antiperspirant is that it is very easy to do, and for the brighter side of it, it can cost you less or nothing at all because they are purely natural, all you need is some certain oil and extracts together with its antibacterial compounds which can add up in removing those unwanted bad smell from your underarm.

Chapter 2 – Artificial Versus Natural Deodorants

Starting with this topic, I'll give you the things you must know in order to understand what is in between these two types of deodorants and how they completely differ from each other. So first things first, what is an artificial deodorant? It is obvious, right?

An artificial deodorant is made up of chemicals and partly natural ingredient. On the other hand, is the All-Natural Deodorant, well we also know that this is very obvious, it all tells it by its name. These deodorants are all made from natural and organic materials or ingredients in order to make those scented anti-bacterial bad odor removing deodorants.Now that I gave you a head start in today's topic, I will be listing down the things you must know why you should switch from artificial deodorant into natural ones. But first why?

In reality, we can use those artificially made deodorants in general but you might want to know that these deodorants don't work at all for some people, because sometimes their body resists these product's effectiveness.

You might be one of these people and in order for you to have a working deodorant product, you might want to try being all-natural in this situation, what I mean is start researching about certain ingredients you can use in making your own natural deodorant that will perfectly work on your body and can adapt on your sweat glands. So now I will be listing down the reasons why you should use natural deodorants than artificial ones.

1. *Artificial deodorants do contain ingredients that can be harmful to your health*

So here we are again talking about the risks of using deodorants and antiperspirants. There is a study that proved, using aluminum-based antiperspirants can increase the chance of having an Alzheimer's disease by 60 percent.

And yet the theory of increasing the chance of having breast cancer by using aluminum-based antiperspirants are here again although this claim about cancer is not yet proven, why not just become safe and try to change your old aluminum-based antiperspirant into a not aluminum based one right?

2. *Natural deodorants have ingredients that are good for your body*

There are natural deodorants that contain charcoal on it, and for you to know, it is not only the natural deodorants that use charcoal but also other cosmetic products. So what does this charcoal do exactly?

It helps absorbs moisture more than you can think of and wait for it, the best part is when charcoal is ingested, it can help you with gastrointestinal problems, can you believe that? Can your recent artificial deodorant do that? There are some plant-based deodorants that can help your underarms to stay fresh and smooth. These ingredients are olive oil, clay-rich in mineral, and Shea butter.

They help make your underarms to become smooth and irritation free. When your underarms do not irritate from the artificial products you use, underarm shaves can last longer. And there are some other ingredients that can help smoothen out razor burns and shrink pores.

The good thing about these natural deodorants is that they don't block the pores in our skin unlike what the antiperspirants do. What these natural deodorant do is they let the good bacteria do their own thing on your skin which is to help lessen the odor.

Because like said previously, it is not the sweat that causes the bad odor, the odor only comes out when the bacteria mixes with your sweat. That's why using natural deodorants can help you get rid of this bacteria, making you smell good.

3. *Does detoxification happen whenever you switch from artificial to natural deodorant?*

There is one statement that said they don't believe in a detoxification period once you switched from artificial to natural deodorant. They stated that once you use the natural one, it will immediately work on the spot.

But for those first timers in using natural deodorants, they must understand that the effectiveness of it still depends on a person's way of living, the food he or she eats and his or her daily physical activities and many more. You must also take note that an aluminum-free deodorant doesn't stop sweat at all.

Those only with ingredients that are safe for you will just help stop the bad odor but they won't keep you dry for the whole day, I mean, they won't keep you dry at all. Just don't stop the sweating, it is not harmful and like said, the sweat is not the one that causes the bad odor, but the bacteria mixed on it. In reality, sweating is a sign that your body is healthy. Don't you want that?

Based on my study, some said that the best way to make the most out of your deodorant is to balance how much you use it. Some people claimed that one or two swipes of deodorants helped them stayed odorless the whole day. And please keep in mind that unlike the artificial deodorants, natural ones only need small amounts to be applied to your underarm in order to work.

Things You Must Know about the Natural and Artificial Deodorants

Of course, you are here for a reason, and that is to know how does these two differ? What are their advantages on each other, disadvantages? And yeah, you are finding the one that will best suit your situation, or in other words, you are finding what product will work best for your body.

It is common for us that we always find precautionary measures in order to be safe from the products that we are going to use.

Well, in this part of the article, I'll be answering down the most common questions asked by people about natural deodorants and artificial deodorants. Stay tuned, you might find the answer you've been looking for here.

1. *Are deodorants and antiperspirants the same?*

For a simpler explanation, the antiperspirants work is to stop the sweat glands from producing sweat, well in reality, not stop at all but reduces its production, while the deodorant, on the other hand, stops that annoying bad odor that lingers around whenever your underarms sweat. Although antiperspirants are also deodorants, not all deodorants are antiperspirants. Think of it as an additional feature for deodorant.

2. *So which one stands out?*

So starting off, antiperspirants stop our sweat glands from sweating right? I believe that you know sweating is a part of the body's process, and it is a sign of healthiness. Sweating is the body's natural way of ventilation. A doctor said that if you don't sweat (naturally), it is a sign that your body can't or doesn't release the toxins inside that can be harmful to us or it is that you are having a bad metabolism.

The aluminum compound in the antiperspirant is an actual aluminum, and it is the most bothering ingredient this product has. So how does this work basically? These small aluminum compounds find their way to block those cells and pores on the skin thus making it look like your sweat glands stopped from producing sweat.

The use of aluminum products like utensils and other stuff has become controversial over the years, and I think that it goes the same with the deodorant. We must stop using aluminum-based antiperspirants. Because long-term use of this aluminum based product can cause serious damage to our tissues.

There is a study that shows aluminum are neurotoxins and can contribute massively to the production of breast cancer cells (the reason why aluminum-based antiperspirants are linked to breast cancer). Not just that, but it can also make the chances of having an Alzheimer's disease high and can cause toxicity in the liver.

Someone said that the use of antiperspirants depends on the person's need. Although the use of antiperspirants is commonly linked with breast cancer, one person stated that the aluminum compounds in the antiperspirants are too small for our body to absorb it completely and cause serious damage inside.

Because studies are still being conducted about the link of antiperspirants on breast cancer, if they are really connected, or if that antiperspirants really cause estrogen to change causing breast cancer cells to increase in amount.

But in order for you to find out what's best for your skin, I suggest that you look at the ingredients of the product you are going to buy.Look if there are common components that can cause skin irritation, these ingredients, for example, are the following propylene glycol, formaldehyde, geraniol, linalool, carboxaldehyde, benzyl salicylate.

And if you are deciding on what type of deodorant to buy, if it's a roll-on, stick, cream or spray. I suggest using the first three and try to avoid sprays, why? Deodorants are meant for skin, not the lungs. It is better to be safe.

3. Any tips on how can I switch from one product to another?

Well, made up your mind already in changing up your old deodorant? But do keep in mind that before starting a new one you must know that it will change your body care routine. Some of the natural deodorant users suggest that you detoxify your underarms first right after you get rid of your old deodorant. And I also believe that this is essential, it is because the detoxification will remove the excess chemicals your old deodorant had left on your underarms.

Think of this as a new fresh start, then right after you've detoxified your underarms, you can now start with your new deodorant brand. There is a simple mask you can make right at your house for this underarm detoxification, all you need is to mix up these ingredients with water: bentonite clay, apple cider, and vinegar.Well if you are not a fan of that detoxification thing, don't worry.

There is a statement that said our body has a natural way of detoxification, and yes I think you already know what that is already. Yes, of course, sweating. Being part of the natural processes of the body, there is no need to worry from chemicals harming you.

When you already started to use your all new natural deodorant and noticed that it is not working at all, you might want to try to exfoliate your underarms once a week. To do these, all you need is a washcloth then mix it up with oat flour and then unscented oil like coconut oil, then you're good to go.

Now that some of your questions are answered, now I will be listing down the reasons why you should avoid artificial deodorants and antiperspirants and start using natural deodorants now. Is it already obvious that all thing that is natural can benefit us a lot than those with chemical. But why do we keep on patronizing this artificial product? Is it because it is easy to buy?

Saves us time in preparing our own because these artificial ones are pre-made already? Yes, these reasons are also beneficial, but come think of this, is it beneficial for your own health? For me, I don't think so.That is why the best way to stay healthy, fresh and odor free, is to get rid of these artificial deodorants and antiperspirants and start using pure natural deodorants and antiperspirants.

Don't mind the time for preparation and the ingredients, because in the end it will be all worth it. So here are the reasons why you should give up your present artificial deodorant and antiperspirant.

1. *Artificial deodorants and antiperspirants contain harmful ingredients*

Yes that is right. It is mentioned a lot in this article, especially the antiperspirant having aluminum on its ingredients. So it is better to stay away from these chemical based products in order to reduce or the best, completely avoid complications in your body.

2. *Natural deodorants don't contain any aluminum*

Although artificial antiperspirants stop the sweat glands from sweating because of the aluminum ions that blocks it. Natural deodorants, on the other hand, work in a very different and safer way. There are compounds in the natural deodorants that help absorb wetness in the underarms effectively, these are plant-based powders and sodium bicarbonate or also known as baking soda.

3. *The scent of natural deodorants are also natural and chemical free*

What does this one mean? Artificial deodorants' scents contain a lot of chemicals in order to create that particular scent.

So imagine now the chemicals that flow right into your body. With the natural deodorants, it is all different, as it provides scent coming from essential oils which are all purely natural.

Chapter 3 – Amazing All-Natural Deodorant Recipes

We are close at the end of this article, and before we part ways, I would like to say thank you for staying until this part, so let us not waste some time, and let's get through this. Now, I will be listing down recipes that can help you make natural deodorants in your own house. I bet that you've read all the things that natural deodorant do? It is all beneficial rather than those artificial ones, right?

And I think that we must be concerned about the products we are using that is why I suggest that you do the natural ones as they don't contain harmful chemicals that artificial deodorants have. There is this ingredient in artificial deodorants called parabens, these include methyl, ethyl, propyl, benzyl, and butyl.

These ingredients are commonly found on the artificial deodorants you are using, and man, that is a lot of chemicals. And there are claims that these chemicals are linked also with breast cancer and other various diseases.

Here are some of the harmful chemicals or ingredients on artificial deodorants that you should avoid:

1. *Parabens (methyl, ethyl, propyl, benzyl, and butyl) - these chemicals are linked with breast cancer and other diseases.*
2. *Aluminum Compounds- often found in antiperspirants, these metallic materials are also linked with breast cancer.*
3. *Silica- These ingredients or chemicals are harmful to the body as they can contribute to cancer and allergies.*
4. *Triclosan- This ingredient is linked with cancer and skin irritations.*
5. *Talc- a chemical that is also linked with cancer.*

6. *Propylene Glycol- these chemicals are linked with liver and kidney problems and also allergic reactions.*
7. *Steareth-n- it is also linked with cancer.*

For the natural deodorant ingredients, here they are:

Homemade Deodorant for a Sensitive Skin

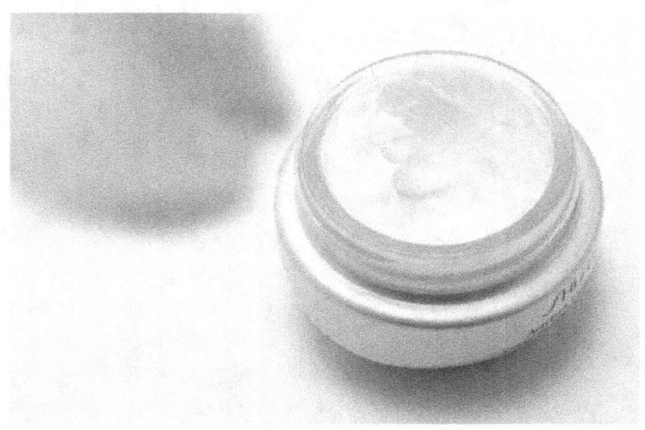

Ingredients:

3/4 cup arrowroot powder/non-GMO cornstarch
1/4 cup baking soda
4-6 tbsp. melted coconut oil

Procedure:

1. In a bowl, mix up the baking soda cornstarch or arrowroot powder
2. Then add up four tablespoons of melted coconut oil then mix. Keep on adding coconut oil until desired consistency is achieved.
3. Put the mixture into a jar with a tight cover.

Shea Butter Deodorant

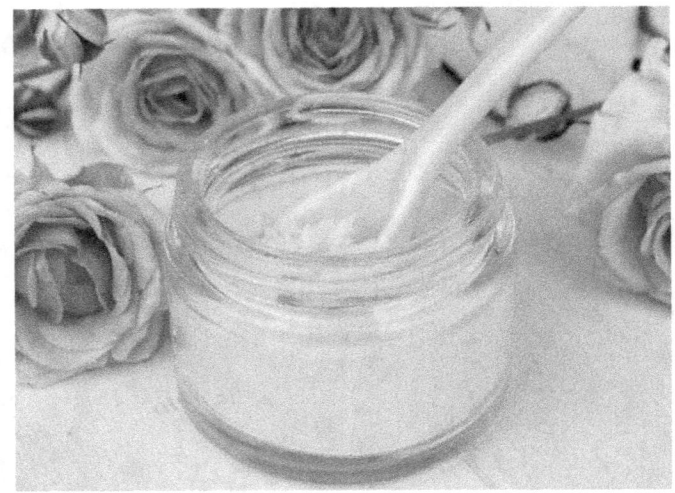

Ingredients:

3 tbsp. coconut oil

3 tbsp. baking soda

2 tbsp. shea butter

2 tbsp. arrowroot (optional) or organic cornstarch

Essential oils (optional)

Procedure:

1. Start by melting the Shea butter and coconut oil in a boiler over medium heat or you can just combine the coconut oil and the Shea butter in a glass jar with a cover then place it over in a pan with water until it melts.
2. Remove from heat then add up the arrowroot or if you don't have arrowroot, add more baking soda.
3. Then add up the essential oils then put all the mixture in a glass container. Don't need to the refrigerator. But it is up to you if you want to put it in the fridge, just to make it hard quickly.

Essential Oil Deodorant

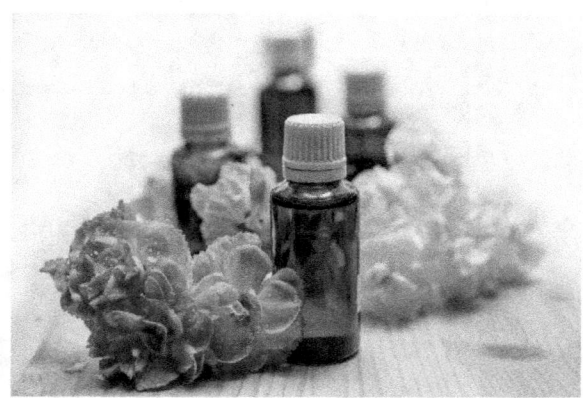

Ingredients:

2 1/2 tbsp. unrefined coconut oil

2 1/2 tbsp. unrefined shea butter

1/4 cup arrowroot starch/flour

2 tbsp. baking soda

6 drops lavender essential oil

6 drops grapefruit essential oil

2 drops tea tree essential oil (optional)

Procedure:

1. In a bowl or jar, put the coconut oil and Shea butter then place the bowl or jar in a medium pan.
2. Add water to the pan, just the right amount to surround the jar or bowl then boil it.
3. As it boils, continue to stir the coconut oil and Shea butter until it melts down.
4. Then right after, place it in separate jars (it is up to you what size) then put it in the fridge so that it will become hard quickly.
5. Make sure to keep the cover on when not in use.

Herbal Deodorant Spray

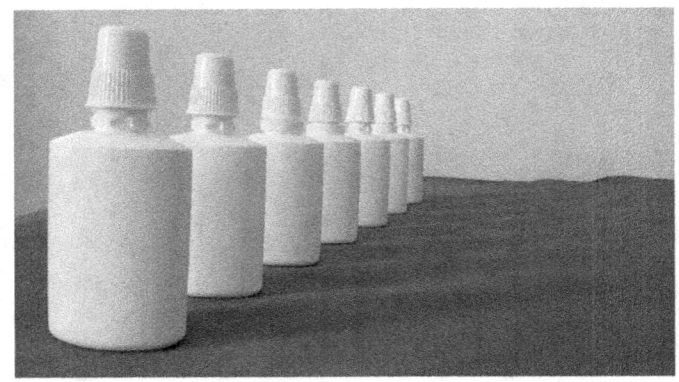

Ingredients:

1¼ cup 80 proof vodka

¼ cup sage leaves

¼ cup thyme leaves

¼ cup lavender buds

Peel of 1 lime or lemon

Essential oils:

Sage (6 drops)

Lavender (4 drops)

Tea tree (3 drops)

Patchouli (3 drops), and either lemongrass or lime(3 drops) per quarter-cup spray bottle

½ tsp. colloidal silver per quarter cup spray bottle, optional

Procedure:

1. In a pint-size jar, measure the herbs and citrus peels.
2. Pour vodka then cover it.
3. Keep the jar in a place where you can always find it, shake it once a day for about a month.

4. When the mixture is ready, funnel the liquid into a spray bottle.
5. Then add up the essential oil for fragrance.
6. Place the drained herbs somewhere you can find it until you are ready to use it again for another mixture.
7. Shake the spray bottle to mix up all the ingredients inside and not letting it only sit right on the top of the bottle.
8. Then you are good to go.

We've come the end of this article and I hope that you've learned a lot about deodorants and antiperspirants. This should give you the knowledge on what to use and how to use them.

To summarize them all, there are certain chemicals found in the ingredients of artificial deodorants and antiperspirants that can be extremely harmful to your health. So it is better to use the artificial ones as they give you the same results in a more safe way and much better.

Conclusion

There you have it, I hope that you have learned a lot from the wonderful deodorant recipes that are included in this book. Do not delay the action now and stop using artificial deodorants and starting switching to the natural ones that are included in the recipes that I mentioned on the previous chapters.

We therefore conclude that those recipes will bring us hundred folds of benefits that is why it is really necessary to put it on your daily routines. Be like me, because based on experience those recipes really improved myself not only my body odor, health, but also my confidence.

So if you want to improve your life for the better then take an action now. I wish you all the best in life!

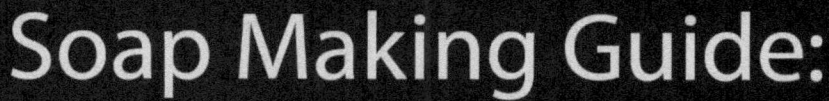

Soap Making Guide:

Beginner's Guide
To Making All-Natural, Mild Soap

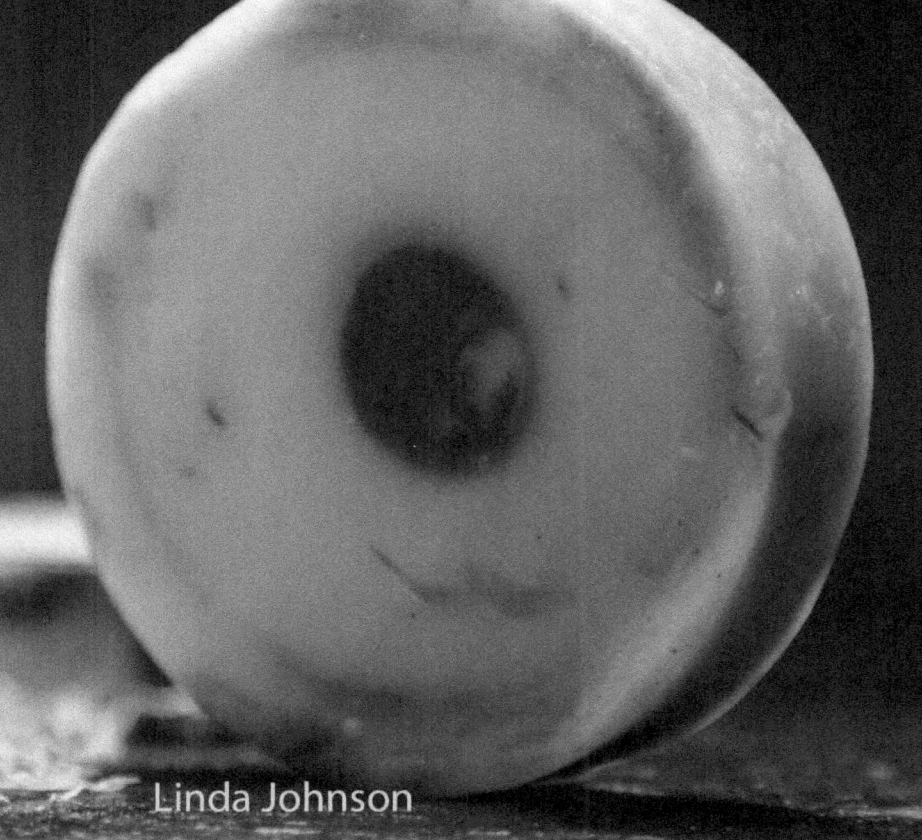

Linda Johnson

Soap Making Guide:

Beginner's Guide To Making All-Natural, Mild Soap

Introduction:

To give you a background about myself the journey of making soap is not that easy because I do not have the proper training in creating soaps beforehand that's why I urged myself to study and practice the craft tremendously until I mastered it. As time passes by, because of training and continued study on the craft I mastered it and in this book I will impart my knowledge to you regarding homemade soap making.

I realized that the knowledge must be shared because I have experienced a lot of benefits from it. Here are the following benefits that I got when I started using the soaps that I created:

- It made my skin smoother because the ingredients are all-natural which will not impose any risks on human's skin.

- My overall health significantly improved and I became more energized by using those soaps.

- Whenever I have a dilemma regarding my skin I just produce a particular soap that will help me solve the problem.

- I save a significant amount of money from buying soaps that I need on various purposes.

Chapter 1 – Different Kinds of Soaps

This is the thing we always use, what I mean is, this thing became part of our daily lives that some of us can't live without it. Can you believe that???! But yes it is true, soaps came from way back the 2800 BC, heck that was a long time ago! Soaps usually consist of natural oils mixed with sodium hydroxide and alkali, these ingredients are the reason why the soaps can clean our bodies effectively, leaving our skin a lot smoother.

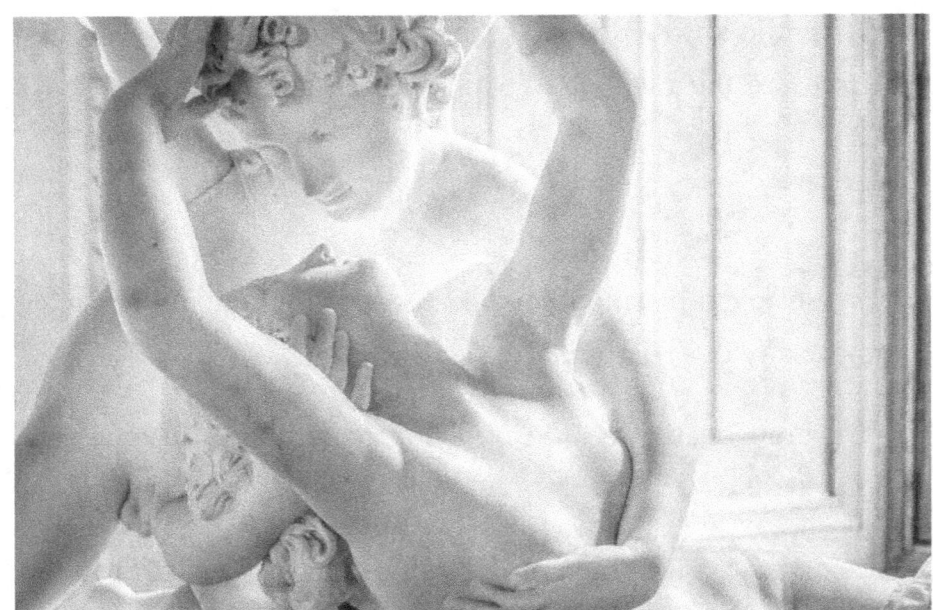

Soaps have different types, they vary in color, scent and the ingredients found on it. These soaps have their own uses and purpose. Like for example, detergents, they are obviously used in cleaning clothes and fabrics. Another one is the dishwashing soap, they are used on cleaning the plates and other utensils at our homes. And there are many more types of soaps with a wide range of use.

Different Kinds of Soaps:

I am sure that there are some of you with a curious mind asks a lot of question, especially about the soap you use. That is why you are here, reading this article. Now I will list down the different kinds of soaps, they're using and how they are made.

- *Toilet Soaps*

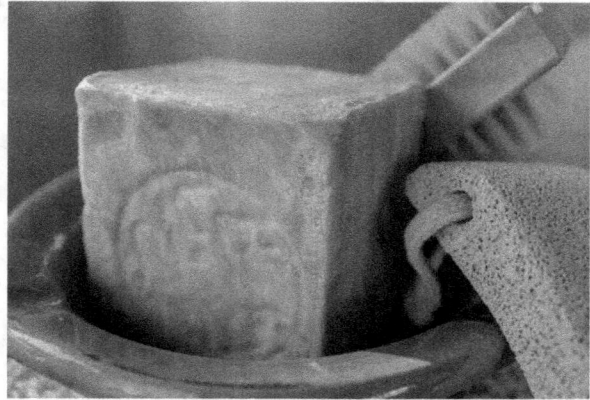

Toilet soaps are the kinds of soaps that are used cosmetically. Toilet soaps are different from bathing soaps, why? Because Totally Fatty Matter or TFM in toilet soaps are large in numbers while on bathing soaps they are low. If the TFM is higher, that only means it is more effective in cleaning. Toilet soaps are divided into three grades.

The first grade contains TFM for about 76%, these soaps are high in quality and they have various colors and scents. The second grade contains TFM for about 70%, these soaps are often smooth and they are commonly white in color. The third grade contains TFM for about 60%, these soaps also have smooth texture on it. But they are commonly red in color due to the acidic content they have. Now knowing all about the grades and some knowledge about the toilet soaps, now I'll be listing down its different kinds.

- *Laundry Soaps*

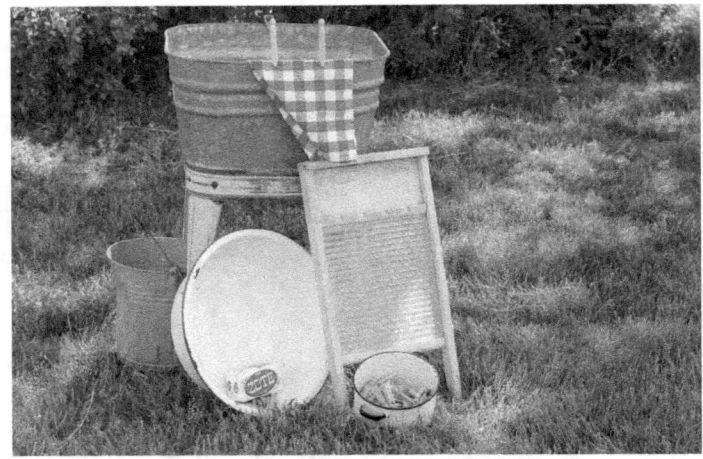

These kind of soaps are the ones we usually see in laundries (well obviously). They can be distinguished as liquid soaps and detergents. The most common ingredient found in a detergent is called surfactant. But you must know that the ingredients every detergent have still varied depending on the brand. There are various ingredients specially used for scents and other characteristics these detergents have. Going back to the surfactant, this ingredient is an active agent.

Surfactants are highly attracted to dirt and water that is why when you use the detergent on laundry, these surfactants attach to the dirt on the clothes and with the help of the water, it pushes the dirt and water upwards to the surface removing the dirt completely from the clothes.

- *Dish Soaps*

Dish soaps are commonly seen as thick liquefied soaps which you need to mix with water in order to use it or sometimes they come in water-based appearance. The ingredients we can commonly see on dish soaps are mint and lemon, why? Is it because they can help easily remove stains from plates and utensils, especially when mixed with warm water.

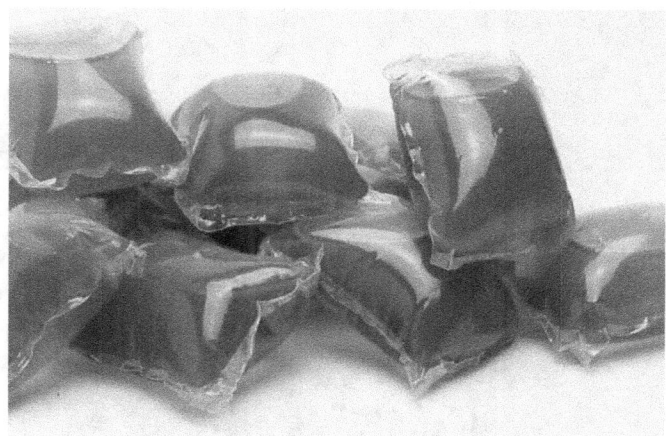

While you scrub the plate with a sponge, this iconic duo (the sponge and the dish soap) will help remove the oils and other unwanted materials from the plates, leaving them on the water's surface ready to be disposed of.

- *Guest Soaps*

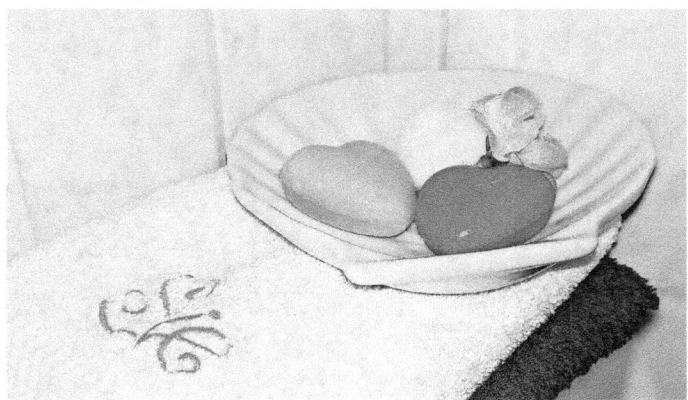

These specific types of soaps are the ones you can see in the hotel rooms. They usually come in small sizes. Imagine them as your standard body cleaning soap. They don't usually have fancy ingredients like essential oils and others. But they do have different scents that you'll like, but remember, bringing them home and stocking them up in place is not recommended. Like said, they are small, that means they usually not last for that long.

- *Beauty Soaps*

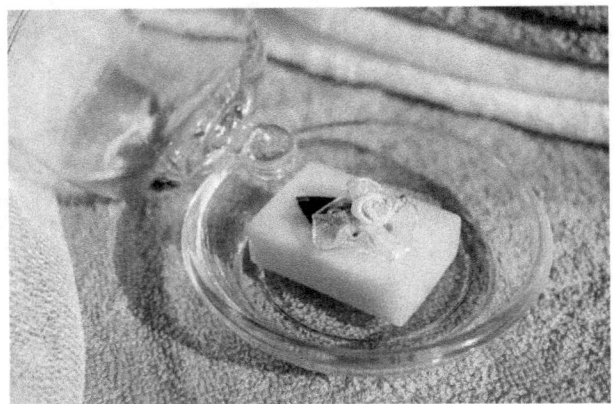

We know that beauty soaps are one of a kind because of the things it offers you, moisturized skin, smooth skin, clearer, and brighter skin and a lot more. There is no doubt that beauty soaps made its way on the top of the kinds of soaps. But be cautious about buying your beauty soaps because not all of them are applicable to your skin. Before buying one, you must know first what skin type you have, then you are good to go. You can choose from the standard bar soaps or the liquefied ones.

- *Medicated Soaps*

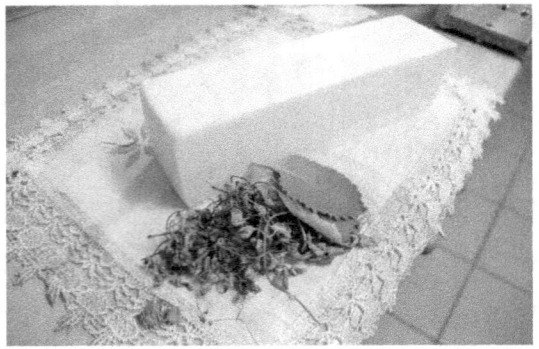

These kinds of soaps are made for one purpose and that is to treat skin diseases and allergies. They help eradicate virus and bacteria from your skin. But the use of medicated soaps is only recommended if the doctor says so.

So all in all, medicated soaps are made with antibacterial ingredients. That is why it is very effective in clearing out your skin off from bacteria and viruses.

- *Novelty Soaps*

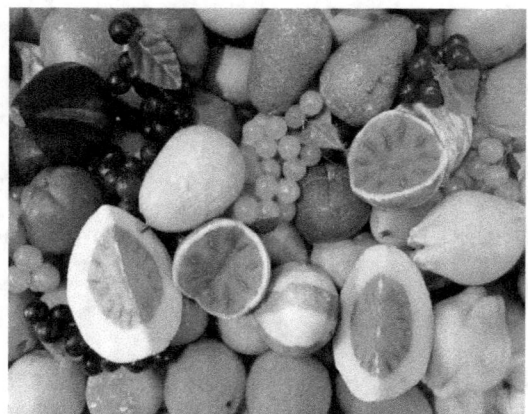

Novelty soaps, they are not your typical soap that cleanses off the germs away. Novelty soap is the kind of soap that is commonly known because of its creative and artistic way of creation. These lovely soaps are best used as gifts for special events like weddings and anniversaries. They are commonly handmade and stands out because of their very soothing fragrance. Well, they may not be your typical soaps, but they can be handy in travels due to their small sizes.

- *Non-Toilet Soaps*

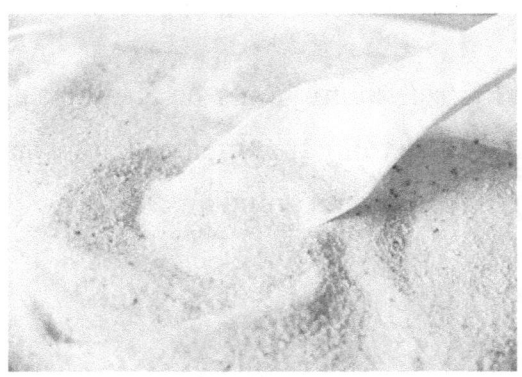

This is the second kind of soap. Well, they are called non-toilet soaps because they are used in heavy cleaning. They are used for removing large amounts of grease and stains. They are not applicable to human skin because they contain acidic ingredients. They are also used as lubricants.

Forms of Soaps (The most common ones)

Of course, if there are different kinds of soap, there will be different forms of it. It may be your standard solid soap or the liquefied ones. So for more information about soaps, I'll be listing down the different forms of soap, the common ones.

Bath Soaps

They appear different from the ones you use in cleaning your whole body while taking a bath and the ones you use just for your face. Bath soaps are generally known for its purpose on making the skin smooth and clean. They can come in bar soaps and sometimes in liquid gels.

Liquid Soaps

The ones we use to buy whenever a bar soap is not available. Liquid soaps are both effective on the whole body and the hands. Also, they are used for the laundry and dishes, one example is the dishwashing liquid.

Liquid soaps have different ingredients or cleaning agents, these depend on the surface they'll be applied on to. The thing that makes liquid soaps stand out from others is that they last longer and easy to bring when going on a travel.

Another thing about liquid soap is that some of them are made of milk, yep you heard that right. These milk soaps are essential for nourishing the skin and making it moisturized and healthy. There are milk soaps used for babies, they are made from goat's milk because goat's milk doesn't contain any harmful elements that can cause irritation on the babies' skin unlike the ones made from artificial materials.

Soaps that gives out good fragrance like the peppermint soap, vanilla soap, seaweed soap and a lot more. These fragrant soaps contain oils that can be found on plants and herbs. These soaps are natural and good for the skin. But apart from others, there are also soaps made out of expensive ingredients or somewhat we can call luxurious. One example are the chocolate soaps (sounds sweet right?), these soaps are made out of cocoa and they can help maintain your skin moisturized.

Bar Soaps

This is the general term for all soap out there (of course I meant for those solid ones and not the liquid versions of them). Bar soaps can be beauty soaps, novelty, laundry or even medicated soaps.

Handmade Soaps

These kind of soaps are by far the safest, why? They are handmade which means they are naturally made, no chemicals added. They are safe for the skin, and what makes these soaps unique is the variety of combinations you can have to create a natural soap.Now you have almost all the knowledge about soaps. So what's next? I bet that you are thinking of creating your own, especially the handmade ones are the safest types right? Don't worry, I got you. I'll be listing down the different methods on how to make soap right at your own home. So what are we waiting for? Let's dive in through this.

Starting with the first method, this is called the "Cold Process Method" (did that just rhyme?). This method is approved and the original one in making soap. So, to start this method, all you need to do is melt down the soft and hard oils together. Then blend it with the lye solution.

But this lye solution and oil solution must be mixed together and melted down with the same temperature, around 90 degrees F. Right after you mixed the two solutions, you need to blend them. This time it is already up to you if you're going to use a blender or you'll blend it manually with a whisk. When properly blended, you can already transfer the mixture into a soap mold. Then you need to cool it down on your fridge for about 4 to 6 weeks before you can put it in action.

The second method is the "Hot Process Method". In this method, the solidification of the soap is much faster, that is why many soap makers really like this method of soap making. To start this method, you're going to melt the oils and mix them with the lye solution. You're going to mix these two mixtures until they become very thick. Then after that, you can pour down the mixture on a soap mold then allow it to cool. When already cooled, you can now use it as a normal soap.

For the third method, it is called the "Room Temperature Method".In this method, all you need to do is gather the hard oils in one container and from there you're going to pour down the hot lye solution. After pouring it, you must stir it gently until the hard oils melt. When the hard oils melt fully, you can now put the soft oils and then blend it all together to form a thick mixture. After creating this mixture, you can now pour it down on a soap mold. Then set it aside for about 4 to 6 weeks like the cold process method before you can use it.

The fourth method is called the "Oven Process Method". This method is actually a general one from the previous three methods. When you are going to use this on the room temperature and cold process methods.

You're going to start on the part where the soap is thick and already poured down on the soap mold, from there you will cook it on the oven for about 150 to 170 degrees F until it becomes gel-like in structure. This method depends on you, some will put the soap molded on the hot oven then turn it off and leave it overnight. And others will cook it for several others. On the other hand, for the hot process method, the oven will be used as the heating device to melt the soap until it becomes thick enough to be poured down on a soap mold.

For the fifth method, it is called the "Whipped Soap Bar Method". This method is quite unique, it doesn't require any heat in order to melt the oils. What you need to do is chill the lye. A soap created using this method has high amounts of hard oils and a few liquid oils. The hard oils in this method are whipped until it becomes thick and soft then the liquid oils will be poured down and blended in. You are going to stir it again and again until it becomes soft and thick like the first mixture.

After achieving this texture, you can now put it in a soap mold then set aside, wait for about 4 to 6 weeks then you're good to go with your homemade soap. The sixth method is called the "Melt and Pour Soap". This method is kinda easy, wait no, actually it is the easiest one because it does not require you to melt down lye solutions and other stuff because it is already premade for you.

What you need to do is just melt this premade lye solution then add your preferred scent and color then pour it right into the soap mold, like the other methods, set aside for weeks then you can use the soap you've just made.

The seventh method is the "Whipped Cream Soap". In this method, you are not making a standard solid soap, but a soap that is soft like whipped cream! This method uses potassium hydroxide and sodium hydroxide and the way to do this one is kind of complicated compared with the other methods listed here. So making this cool soap can take a lot of time and effort.

The eighth method is called the "Glycerin Soap or Transparent Soap". Hence the name, these soaps are transparent. In making a transparent soap, you need to use the hot process method but a little different, when the process reaches on the point of the soap being thick enough, the alcohol and glycerin are now added in order for the soap base to be dissolved.

When the base already melted, on the glycerin solution, there is a sugar solution added in order to help for the transparency of the soap. At this point, you can now add the scent and color of your choice on the mixture. Stir them gently then right after, you can put it now on the soap mold and set it aside for about 4 weeks then you can use your transparent soap. Keep in mind that this step is not that easy because, in some countries, they require you to have this special license in order to buy the alcohol needed for your transparent soap.

For the ninth and last method, it is called the "Liquid Soap Making". Well, in this method, you are making a liquefied soap and this method is the same as the transparent method the only difference is that you don't use sodium hydroxide but you use potassium hydroxide(keep in mind that potassium hydroxide is the main ingredient when making a soft soap or liquid soap).

There are two methods on making liquid soap, they are the alcohol lye method and the paste method. The paste method uses the hot process method until it comes on the procedure's stage of thickening, from there the mixture will be diluted and neutralized then sequestered for weeks.

For the alcohol method, the oils are mixed up with the lye solution, then the alcohol is added then the mixture will be brought to trace. Then right after, the soap will be boiled for hours the same as the paste method, will be diluted and neutralized then sequestered for weeks. To make the most of this method, you should familiarize yourself first with the hot and cold process method.

Chapter 2 – Soap Recipes For Smoother Skin

Ever see a whitening soap or a soap that can make your skin smoother in the mall but you can't afford it? But do you know that you can make these soaps right in your home? Yes, that is right! With the right ingredients, you can make these soaps in no time. They all have the same quality and the best part? The one you make in your home is a lot safer than the commercial ones because of the natural ingredients you'll be using.

Grapefruit Mint Poppy Seed Soap

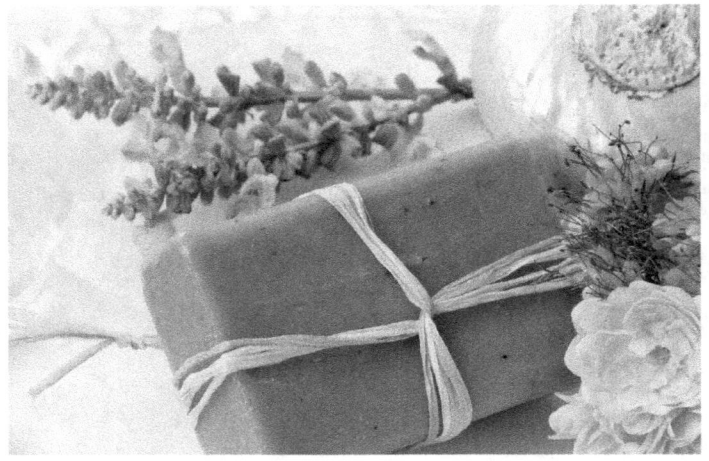

The ingredients you need:

10 oz. <u>goat's milk melt-and-pour soap base</u>
1 grapefruit
1 tbsp. poppy seeds
10 drops of <u>grapefruit essential oil</u>
4 drops of <u>peppermint essential oil</u>

Procedure:

1. Get your goat milk soap base then cut it into cubes.
2. Scrape the grapefruit you have then prepare the poppy seeds.
3. Set your microwave in a standard heating mode or prepare your stove for boiling then melt the soap on either of the two.
4. While it melts, stir it gently. Be careful not to burn the soap.
5. When the soap is already melted, put it in a container where it can fit exactly, then add the grapefruit you've just scraped, the poppy seeds and the oils.
6. Stir the mixture you've just made.
7. Then next is, pour the melted soap mixture on the soap mold then set aside until it gets hard. It will usually take about 2 to 3 hours before it completely hardens.
8. When it is hard already, you can pop them out from the mold and use them (you can also prepare them as gifts).

Aloe Vera Soap

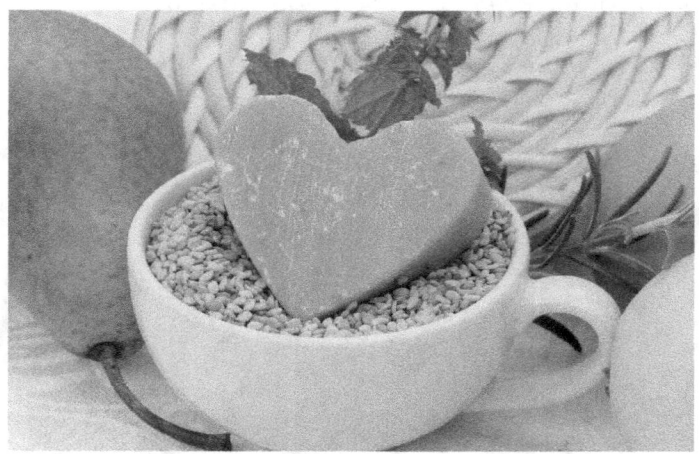

The ingredients you need:

14.9 oz. coconut oil

13.4 oz. olive oil

10.5 oz. <u>lard</u>

2.5 oz. <u>shea butter</u>

9.6 oz. g <u>aloe gel</u> and water purée

6.7 oz. <u>lye (NaOH)</u>

9.9 oz. water

Procedure:

1. On a bowl or any container of your choice, pour the water and add the lye.
2. On a stove or a microwave oven, heat up and melt the oils.
3. When the oil melts, add the lye mixture to the melted oil.
4. Right after adding the lye mixture, add the aloe gel.
5. Mix them well until the mixture becomes thick enough.
6. Pour the mixture on a soap mold and set aside for about a day or two.
7. When it hardens already, you can now use it.

Vanilla Citrus Soap

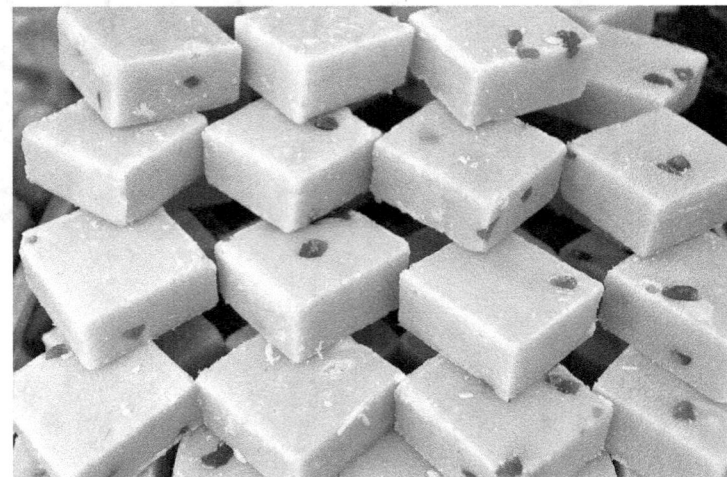

The ingredients you need:

6 small cubes of melt & pour soap base

Vanilla essential oil or extract

Orange peel

Poppy seeds

Silicone Molds

Procedure:

1. Meltdown the small cubes of your soap base in a microwave (be sure to put it on a microwavable bowl).
2. While the soap base on the process of melting, zest the orange peel.
3. When the soap is already melted, remove it from the microwave and prepare it for pouring in the mold.
4. On a bowl, pour down the melted soap base and then add the orange zest, poppy seeds, and the vanilla oil, stir them gently.
5. When they are already mixed up well, carefully pour the mixture on the silicone molds.
6. Set aside for about 2 hours.
7. When they are already hard, you can pop them off from the silicone mold and now ready for use.

Chapter 3 – DIY Germicidal Soap Recipes

A bit more conscious about the soap you use? Of course, the first thing that comes to mind is to buy a soap that can protect you from certain viruses and bacteria that can cause skin allergies. But, like the most soaps, you can make your own antibacterial soap right in your home!

Shea Butter with Coconut Milk Soap

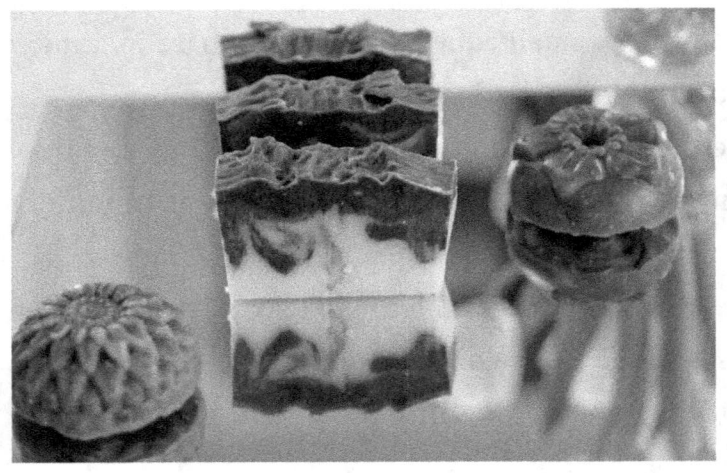

The ingredients you need:

Shea Butter -135 gr.

Coconut Oil -6.35 oz.

Olive Oil -12.7 oz.

Castor Oil - 3.175 oz.

Palm Oil- 4.8 oz.

Distilled Water -7.05 oz.

Coconut Milk -3.42 oz.

Lye -4.34 oz.

Calendula Flower Petals

Procedure:

1. On a pan, warm up the coconut milk and then set it aside.
2. Follow the standard soap making method on making your soap batter (mix the water and lye).
3. Finely mince the Calendula flower petals.
4. Make a thin trace from this soap batter mixture. Then right after add the coconut milk.
5. Stir the mixture gently until it reaches a medium trace.
6. Get your soap mold and then pour down ¾ of the soap batter.
7. On the remaining soap batter, add the Calendula flower petals and stir it well.
8. Then add the remaining soap batter on the mold.
9. Set it aside for about a week until it gets hard.
10. Once hard, you can now pop it off from the soap mold and use it.

Olive Oil Soap

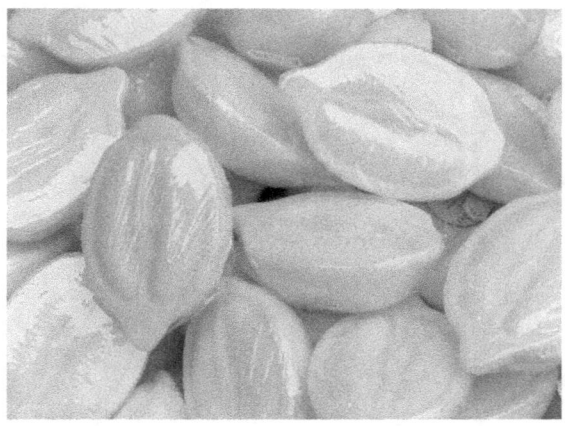

The ingredients you need:

Coconut Oil - 6.35 oz.

Infused Olive Oil - 19.05 oz.

Palm Oil - 6.35 oz.

Distilled Water - 11.5 oz.

Lye - 4.27 oz.

Dried chamomile and calendula

Procedure:

1. To start off in making this antibacterial soap, mix the olive oil and the dried calendula and chamomile.
2. Using a pot, put it on low heat for an hour then right after, set aside and leave overnight.
3. After setting it aside, drain the extract leaving the solid materials.
4. Make the soap mixture by mixing the water and lye.
5. Melt the soap mixture and then add the olive oil mixture on it.
6. When the soap mixture comes into a thin trace, you can now pour it into the soap mold.
7. Set aside for about 4 to 6 weeks and then you can use the soap right after.

Chapter 4 – Colorful Soap Recipes

One thing that makes soap popular in the market is because of its artistic designs. Some soaps are made for decorations, these soaps are called "Novelty Soaps". By having this cool and unique designs on the soap, take note that they are not as effective as an original soap. They can clean but not that much. But don't worry, if you are an artist like me, then let's dive right into making these colorful and unique soaps.

Swirly Soap

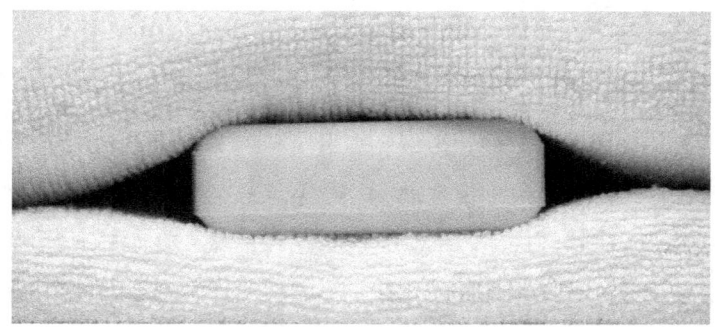

The ingredients you need:

Coconut Oil - 9.52 oz.

Olive Oil - 12.7 oz.

Castor Oil - 1.59 oz.

Palm Oil- 7.94 oz.

Distilled Water - 12.06 oz.

Lye - 129.15 gr.

Cocoa Powder - 1/4 Tsp.

Black Oxide - 1/4 Tsp.

Yellow Oxide - 1/4 Tsp.

White Mica - 1 1/4 Tsp.

Procedure:

1. By doing this recipe, you need to follow the "Room Temperature Method" recently discussed.
2. Mix the oils, water, and the lye to make the soap mixture.
3. Mix the soap mixture on a warm heat until it reaches a thin trace.
4. After reaching a thin trace, get a soap mold with four molds on it (you're going to use these four spaces for the colors).
5. Pour the soup mixture on the soap mold (equally divided on the four molds).
6. One by one, add each color on each of the four molds.
7. Mix them gently.
8. Grab another soap mold.
9. On the other soap mold, drizzle down one soap color then add the other three (drizzle it on a swirling pattern).
10. When they are all mixed up and swirled, you can now set aside the soap to make it hard.
11. Once the soap hardens, you can now pop it off from the soap mold and use it, or gift wrap it and use it as a gift for a friend or relative on a special event.

Coffee Soap

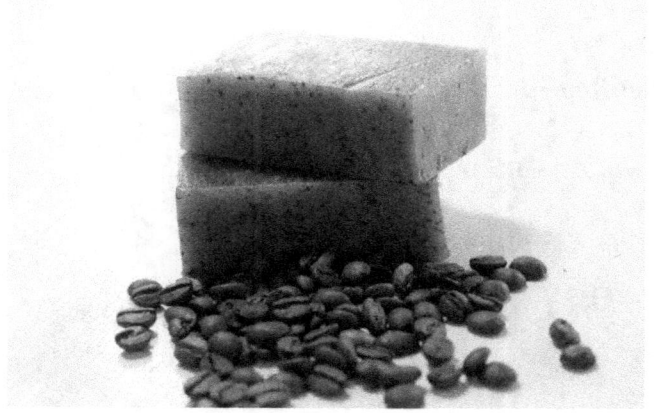

The ingredients you need:

Shea Butter - 135 gr.

Coconut Oil - 7.9 oz.

Olive Oil - 11.1 oz.

Castor Oil - 3.18 oz.

Palm Oil - 4.76 oz.

Distilled Water - 324 gr.

Lye - 125.25 gr.

Essential Oils of Ginger - 1/2 tsp.

Essential Oils of Cinnamon - 1/2 tsp.

Essential Oils of Clove - 1/2 Tsp.

Essential Oils of Patchouli- 1/2 Tsp.

Essential Oils of Sweet Orange - 6 Tsp.

Finely Ground Oatmeal - 2 Tbsp.

Cocoa Powder - 1 tsp.

Finely ground coffee - 1 Tbsp.

Confectioners' Sugar - 1 tsp.

Orris Root Powder - 1 tsp.

Procedure:

1. Prepare the oils, the water and the lye. On this part of the procedure, it is up to you on what soap making method you are going to use.
2. Once the soap mixture is created. Stir it until it reaches a thin trace.
3. After reaching a thin trace, pour ¼ of the soap mixture into the soap mold.
4. Right there, add the cocoa powder, ground coffee, Orris root powder, ground oatmeal and sugar, mix them well.
5. Pour down all the essential oils on the mixture and mix them quickly.
6. Then you can now set it aside.
7. When it is hard already, you can now use it or make it as a gift for someone special.

Chapter 5 – Creative Multipurpose Soap Recipes

The large variety of soaps have their own purpose. But what if you can have a soap that is antibacterial and at the same time a beauty soap? Isn't that convenient for you? But sadly, some of these high-quality multipurpose soaps are expensive in the market but don't you worry, I'll be helping you on making your own multipurpose soap right in your own home. So what are you waiting for? Let's start with the first multipurpose soap recipe.

Anise Soap

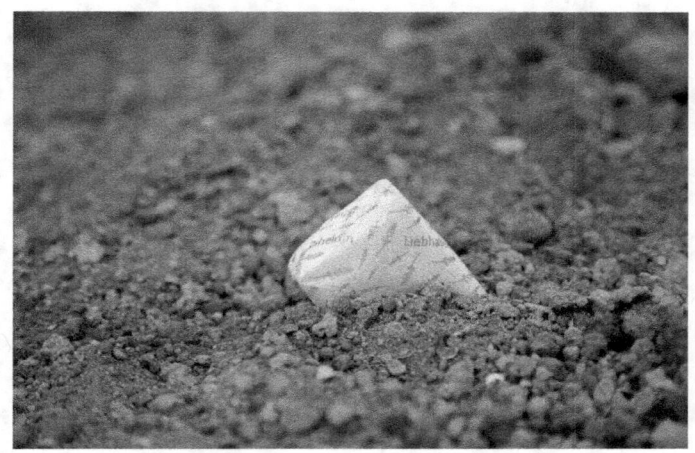

The ingredients you need:

Shea Butter - 45 gr.

Coconut Oil - 7.937 oz.

Olive Oil - 11.11 oz.

Castor Oil - 1.587 oz.

Palm Oil - 9.524 oz.

Distilled Water - 6.31 oz.

Coconut Milk - 3.53 oz.

Lye - 127.05 gr.

Essential Oils of Anise - 1/2 Tsp.

Essential Oils of Sweet Fennel - 1/2 Tsp.

Essential Oils of Sweet Orange - 2 Tsp.

Essential Oils of Cinnamon - 1/4 tsp.

Essential Oils of Clove Bud - 1/4 Tsp.

Essential Oils of Nutmeg - 1/4 tsp.

Rose Fragrance Oil - 4 Tsp.

White Mica - 1 Tsp.

Black Oxide - 1/2 Tsp.

Orris Root Powder - 1 Tsp.

Procedure:

1. In this soap recipe, it is also up to you on what soap making method you are going to use.
2. Once you've picked your preferred soap making method, start by mixing the shea butter, coconut oil, olive oil, palm oil, castor oil, water, and the lye on a bowl or a container where they can all fit.
3. When already mixed, you've just made your soap mixture.
4. Continue mixing the mixture until it comes into a thin trace.
5. When it reaches the thin trace, add the coconut milk, white mica, Orris root powder, the rose fragrance scent, and the black oxide.
6. Stir the mixture well until it reaches a medium trace.

7. When already on medium trace, you can now pour down the mixture on the soap mold.

8. Finish the procedure based on the soap making method you've chosen.

Matcha Soap

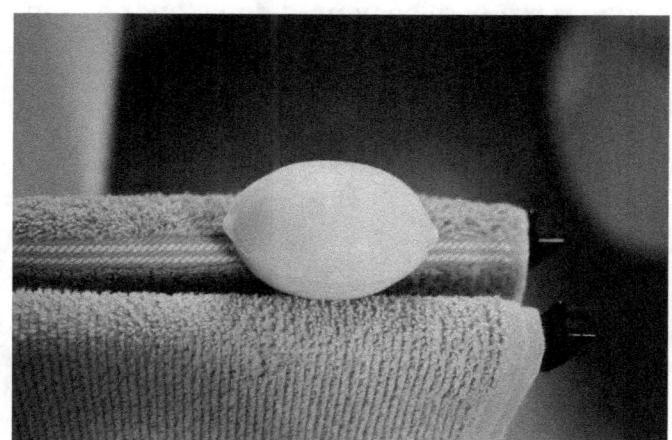

The ingredients you need:

1 pound melt & pour glycerin soap

2 tbsp. matcha powder

3/4 tsp. lemon essential oil

Soap Mold

Procedure:

1. Slice the 1 pound melt and pour the soap into small pieces and put them in a microwavable bowl.

2. Set the microwave to high heat and then put the bowl with the soap inside.

3. Let it sit there for about 30 seconds.

4. After that, get the bowl and stir it gently then put it back on the microwave for about 15 seconds or 20 seconds.

5. After that, get the bowl out of the microwave and then stir again.

6. Repeat step 4 and 5 until the soap melts completely.

7. When the soap already melts, get it out of the microwave and then add the matcha powder and the lemon essential oil. Stir well.

8. Now the soap is ready to be poured down on the soap mold.

9. After putting it on the soap mold, you can now let it sit for about a week before you can use it.

Cream Soap

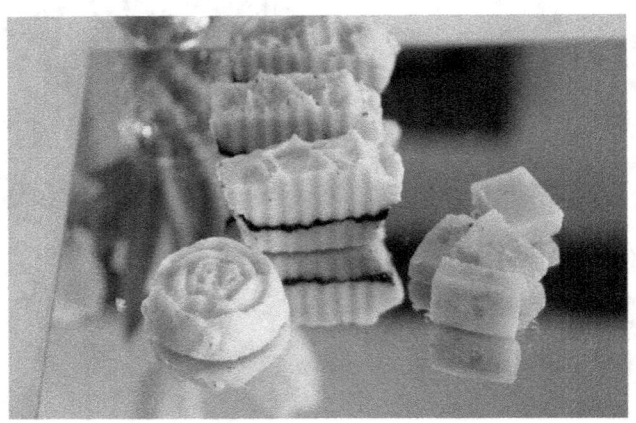

The ingredients you need:

1 bar soap

4-6 cups water

1 tsp. Glycerin

2 cups vegetable shortening

1 cup of coconut oil

10-15 drops essential oils (optional)

Procedure:

1. Start by shredding the bar of soap, after shredding it, set the soap aside.
2. Prepare your stove to medium heat and then on a pot, put the shredded soap and add 4 cups of water. Let it sit on medium heat for about 30 minutes.
3. After the 30 minutes time interval, add the glycerin on the melted soap, stir it well.
4. Pour down the mixture of the soap and glycerin on Styrofoam cups and let it cool.
5. You'll notice that the soap will slowly turn thick.
6. Put the soap on a bowl and let it cool again.
7. As the soap is in the process of cooling down, start making the whip.
8. Grab a large bowl, and there, add the coconut oil and the vegetable shortening.
9. Mix these two ingredients until it becomes thick.
10. When it becomes thick already, you can now add the cooled down soap.
11. Whip the soap and the mixture until it turns into a whipped cream texture.
12. Add the optional essential oil then you're good to go.

Peppermint Soap

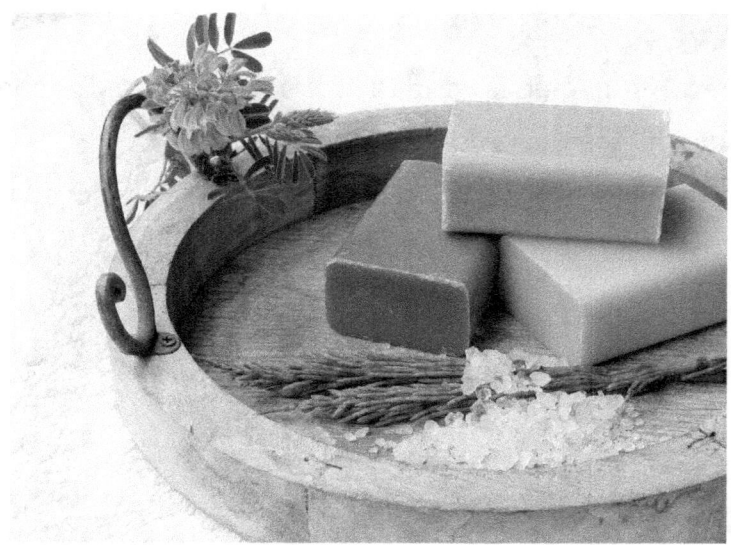

The ingredients you need:

2 lbs. <u>Shea butter melt and pour soap</u>

Peppermint Oil

1 box Crushed Candy Canes

Rubbing Alcohol in a spray bottle

Soap Mold

Procedure:

1. On a pot, melt down the shea butter and pour soap for about an hour.
2. When the shea butter and the soap already melt, add about 10 to 12 drops of peppermint oil, mix well.
3. Prepare the soap mold, spray it with rubbing alcohol so that bubbles from the soap will not be created.
4. Now pour the melted soap on the soap mold then add the crushed candy canes on the top.
5. The next thing to do is wrap the soap and let it sit for about 2 hours so that it will not dry out while in the process of hardening.
6. When the soap is already hard, you can now use it or wrap it as a gift.

Conclusion

So if you want to take your life to the next level and make something new out of your creativity then you can make use of the soap recipes that we have discussed. Once you mastered this lovely soap making craft, you can modify the ingredients and shapes according to your own preferences.

I hope that you have learned a lot from this book and I am looking forward to your growth no matter what plan do you have in your new craft whether you will just use it for your own personal use or make it as a business it's up for you to decide.

www.ingramcontent.com/pod-product-compliance
Lightning Source LLC
Chambersburg PA
CBHW052040280526
45791CB00010B/3026